The Quest
Healing Journal

Give a Gift that Makes a Difference...

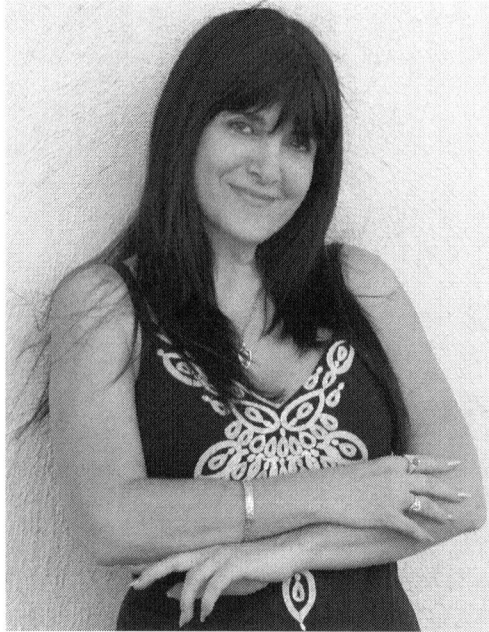

My prayer is that TheQuest Self Healing System
finds everyone it is meant for
so that lives,
families and communities
around the world can be healed.

Please Support the Institute of Advanced Healing's Global Outreach Program

Your Tax Deductible donations gift TheQuest Self Healing System to prisons, rehab centers, hospitals, hospice, safe houses, youth at risk, PTSD, abuse, anger management, and addiction programs, or the designation of your choice in your name.

Donate & Find out more at:
http://www.AuroraJulianaAriel.com,
http://www.IOAH.org, or http://www.TheQuest.us

Thank you for helping me bring TheQuest to the world.

Aurora Juliana Ariel

Praise for TheQuest

Jack Canfield, author of 'Success Principles' and co-author of the 'Chicken Soup for the Soul' Series: TheQuest session with Aurora was a magical and helpful experience. It unblocked a subtle but powerful limitation in my life. I am grateful to her for her work and for her safe and gentle way of being.

Jared Rosen, Co-Author of 'The Flip' and, 'Inner Security And Infinite Wealth': TheQuest is a ratified healing system that works at such a core level, that ancient subconscious patterns clear at lightning speed. Aurora is truly a master!

Randolph Craft, founder, Pacific Planning Institute, and Pacific International Aging Center: The space Aurora holds for healing is so powerful that one has no choice but to move forward in her Presence.

Aeoliah, Author, Artist, Composer, Recording Artist: I was pleasantly surprised to find Aurora's TheQuest work to be so simple and straightforward, yet at the same time so dynamic and powerful in helping to shift deep-seated limiting energy patterns hidden within my subconscious. I found it to be a most healing experience to give a voice to my deeper feelings and express how I really felt about certain things in my life in a supportive, caring and non-judgmental setting that helped me to transform those patterns into the fulfillment that I desire. During the session I also enjoyed and appreciated the balance between voicing and openly expressing my feelings, and then later tuning into my Higher Self to allow and receive the messages from my own God Presence which made the experience my own personal empowerment that I cherish in my heart forever.

A Physical Therapist and former Christian Evangelist in California: The diminishment of the human condition is based on lack of self worth and esteem, and no amount of verbal affirmation will transform us. It has to come from an Alchemy within. In TheQuest sessions, the very molecules are rearranged, as cells not nourished are now nourished from within. We are truly cleansed from this inner work. This is like a soul clean up, or 50,000 mile check up for the inner being. The best part is that the changes are permanent. I can't believe how changed I am. People notice a calm and clarity. I have not reverted to the pattern since our last session. I cannot think of a better birthday gift than a chance to heal the inner soul of the grief and debris from our years before. —*D.J. Martinovich, Physical Therapist, Palm Springs, California*

Christopher Connolly, Composer, Recording Artist: Dr. Aurora Juliana Ariel's abilities as a Healer are so remarkable it is hard to put into words. My work with her was so profoundly deeply moving and transformational that I felt as if I had literally been bathed in the serene waters of the Holy Spirit. Her voice and presence guided me to a Divine place of Inner Peace.

A former nurse manager in Wisconsin: TheQuest process is awesome. I have been through a lot of counseling since the age of 18. I knew as an adult child of alcoholics, without a good role model, I was going to need guidance to overcome my past even at that young age. As a nurse, I have also been exposed to mental heath treatment methods in my career. I have never experienced anything as impressive and empowering. Aurora is a wonderful, loving person who creates a safe space for the deepest healing. —*Virginia Furumo, who is now living her dream life in Hawaii*

Michele Gold, Author of 'Angels of the Sea', Artist and Musician: I had been feeling very sad, almost hopeless, which is very unlike my Nature, for quite awhile, and within 24 hours of my TheQuest Counseling session with Aurora, it just lifted. Nothing outwardly changed and yet, I felt happy inside, a peace with where I was at. It was huge. Aurora's healing gifts are very powerful! The energy that had been suppressed inside me came forward and new projects began moving and many new creative ideas were bursting forth. I felt freer than I had felt in many years, happier, and filled with a quiet confidence that was battered for so long, and now was emerging from an ancient cocoon, with new shimmering wings with which to soar. Aurora Juliana Ariel is a rare radiant treasure. Her magnificent alchemical gifts will embrace you and guide you in a manner filled with so much love and compassion, you will feel free, your most profound self validated to emerge and shine. To experience Aurora's powerful healing work is to sit in the center of an exquisite circle of angels, supporting your soul's deepest wish to transform and live the most exceptional, magical life you were born to live.

Kamala Allen, PhD, Author of 'A Woman's Guide to Opening a Man's Heart': Aurora Juliana Ariel channels Mother Mary energy in an atmosphere of unconditional love and profound peace. Her gentle, effective approach to healing is a deep experience of nurturance and transformation.

A Police Officer and High School Teacher in Aspen: Dr. Ariel's method of going inside one's self and healing past issues or gaining self-realizations is really quite amazingly simple, yet very valuable. Almost like finding a key to a hidden treasure. In Dr. Ariel's presentation to my class at Aspen High School, I got to see a side of Aurora that impresses me to no end. Both the spiritual side, but also the vulnerable sharing and compassionate side that has such great love, desire, energy, and compassion to help the world and a great mind to go with all that. She really connected to the kids and I guarantee that is not an easy thing to do these days. She will make a difference and I feel very fortunate I somehow was blessed I got to meet her. My hat's off to her in a big way. —*Brad Onsgard, Aspen High School Teacher and Law Enforcement Officer*

A Youth Zone Counselor: When meeting with a court-ordered youth, I noticed an enormous shift in his attitude and responsibility in a very short period of time... So I asked him "What has happened to cause you to mature so quickly?" That's when he told me that he was in a program for teens (TheQuest Teen Forum) that was making a huge difference for him. While he still has a way to go in his life, I have not seen such a huge internal shift in a youth like this in a very long time. My interest in the TheQuest came from seeing results, not from hearing about the program. Fantastic work! — *Shawn Stevenson, MSW, Youth At Risk Counselor, Case Manager for Youth Zone*

A teen in Hawaii: TheQuest is a great way to get things off your chest and deal with feelings that have been deep inside and yet are effecting us in a negative way. It really works! —*Aradeus Zachariah Daffin, 16 years old, Maui, Hawaii (Dr. Ariel's youngest son, now 21, received TheQuest Master Counselor Training with Dr. Ariel for 18 months and co-facilitated the first TheQuest Teen Forum with her in Aspen)*

A mother of an angry, violent eight-year-old: My daughter is doing really well! Thank you so much for working with her, I can really tell a difference in her self-esteem and overall well-being. I can see she really feels great about her appointments with you! After two sessions, three teachers called and asked what happened to her, she had changed so much! Namaste. —*Kelly Sundstrum, Carbondale, Colorado*

A mother whose son was traumatized by a fatal accident where he was the driver: Aurora, you are our angel. You accomplished in five days what doctors and other professionals around us believed would take 8 months for my son to fully recover and get to. Being with you this short time, my son is a changed person. I am very grateful! —*Patti S., Colorado Springs, Colorado*

And others....

Aurora's mastery shines as she navigates us through the terrain of our soul, allowing all of our self to be seen and expressed, thus granting greater freedom, wisdom, and insight. With her keenly trained mind, she lovingly and compassionately guides us in and through the closed doors and murky waters of our unexpressed parts, revealing hidden resources that bring solutions to our every day life, catalyzing deep awakening and a greater understanding of our self. —*Rev. Adrianna Levinson, Vibrant Life Center, Maui, Hawaii*

I had pronated knees since I was a little girl. Continually aggravating the condition through a very active and full life, it became a life long affliction. By 25 years old I had to stop running, a great passion in my life! I also loved to ski, hike, and bike, but my knees would get so sore that my lifestyle was greatly hindered. At TheQuest Life Mastery Training Course in Aspen, I had the opportunity to work with Dr. Ariel. In my session we traced a pattern back to early childhood where I had suffered severe abuse. As we unlocked and healed the pattern, I felt a tremendous release. The very next day I was working out at the Aspen Club gym when, looking in the mirror, I noticed my legs were straight. My trainer came over and could hardly believe his eyes. The condition was healed! —*Diane Argenzio, Estate Manager, Aspen, Colorado*

After years of being in and out of therapy I had changed my life very little but after four Counseling sessions with Aurora I was a new person. I had come to the first session a skeptic, but by the time we were done I was totally amazed by the amount of healing that took place. I had been hitting my head against the wall not getting any movement in my years of therapy. Traditional therapy had only scratched the surface, whereas TheQuest dove right into the root of the issue, uncovered the truth, and healed that aspect of my inner self. The sessions have been the most powerful events in my life. I'm finally free of the unhealthy part of myself that was holding me back for years. I never thought transformation like this was truly possible. I'm no longer a victim of the past and my emotional traumas have been set free. I have my life back! I made more progress in a few sessions with Dr. Ariel than I had in years of therapy. Since we worked together, a lot changed in my life. I married the woman of my dreams and it has only gotten better. Now we have a little daughter. This was all made possible because of Dr. Ariel and TheQuest work. Thank you, Dr. Ariel from the bottom of my growing heart!—*Lance Koberlein, Programmer Real Estate Broker Entrepreneur, Denver, Colorado*

Gone are the days of long drawn out traditional therapies! With Aurora's 'TheQuest' work, I have found a way to heal and transform any pattern or history from ancient to present times. The space she creates in her sessions is nurturing, loving, empowering and safe. I have found a new sense of purpose in life with each healing of the darker aspects of myself, a greater love for all that I am. TheQuest allows me to address issues as they come up and access the core of the issue to transform it all in one session! I am so grateful for Aurora's dedication to the healing arts and her loving presence, which has empowered me as a wife, mother, businesswoman, healer, and human being. —*Colleen Lisowski, Business Owner/ Healer, Kula, Hawaii*

Since the session I have a very clear mind, not used to it. All energy is there and the creativity is fully able to explode into any direction it needs to without any interruption. Wow! Still settling in the experience and taking apart the system for a deeper grasp and understanding. —*Arben Kryeziu, Business, Marketing, and Internet Consultant*

My heart is so open and full from this work. Being gently led through the deepest, darkest places leaves only gratitude, love and freedom. In every session we come quickly to the taproot of the issue, create safety for its exposure and transformation, and watch the magic with awe as the entire tree is healed. Aurora's work embodies the violet flame. Transformation and healing occur in her presence. She is a miracle as is every experience I have with her. Colors are brighter, scents are sweeter, sounds are crisper, air is clearer. Working with Aurora is like buying a shuttle pass to Heaven. The entire experience of being human is a greater joy as a result of these clearings.

This work helps me feel so purposeful; proud to be a human, finally. The tools that Aurora uses for healing are pure magic, like laser surgery for the soul. The operation is fast, relatively painless and totally effective. People would not choose to live with pain if they knew this was available. Miracles with Aurora are commonplace. In every session I have the experience that something very profound has taken place, something life changing of a permanent nature. The power of love to heal used to be an expression. After working with Aurora it is a fact. This gentle, precise soul surgeon is a master at healing. —*Miriam Mara, Business Consultant, Boca Raton, Florida*

I feel differently. My attitude has changed. I definitely have transcended my pattern. I am a whole new being! TheQuest session was like an exorcism, casting a demon out of my being that was like a leach, sucking the life force out of me, and preventing me from being who I am as a person. After one session, I am a completely different person. —*Bruce Travis, Author, Real Estate Broker, Wailea, Hawaii*

After 20 years of being intimately involved in the human potential movement, reading endless material, attending every conference I could, listening to speakers, reading their books, and applying their principles, I was never taken to the places I was told they would take me. They just didn't hold up and I would soon be back into my old patterns without knowing why things were not working for me. Then I met Aurora and started receiving TheQuest sessions. Right away, after the 1st session, I realized there was a deeper place I needed to go to resolve the issues in my life. I learned of the importance of finding the root of the problem instead of adopting a philosophy which doesn't eliminate the effect things have had on my life. My life has changed considerably with the elimination of stress, eliminating guilt and frustration, and knowing I can be completely honest with myself and those around me. My self-esteem has been restored to a new high. Each day I look forward to meeting new people, making friends, creating relationships, and enjoying new, and exciting experiences. There is a new outlook on life that has never been there before, and I am free to achieve my goals and aspirations. I am so grateful for this life changing experience of TheQuest. —*Bill Mollring, Business Owner*

Aurora brings a special presence to her work as higher energies work through her causing transformation for the individual. I have personally experienced this and have benefited by releasing, clearing, and transforming at a very deep level. Experiencing her work has helped me to take my own healing work to a deeper and more powerful level. —*Lisbeth Johnson, Certified Rolfer, Columbus, Ohio*

I went from panic to peace in my session. It was incredible. Through this work, I'm feeling a new sense of well being. Everything is shifting. Sometimes I don't even recognize this new person. I am healing after 57 years in life, finally getting 'it' with the help of my guide, Dr. Ariel. —*Kamalia Vonlixfeld, Owner, Lotus Galleries, Kauai*
The session was incredible! I am so much less fearful. Even though it seems that nothing

has changed in the physical, I see things differently. —*Mary Miller, Editor*

My life is very changed. I am showing up differently in my relationship with my husband, my son and others. TheQuest has brought me a renewed sense of faith in the Divine. —*DB. Healer/Mother, Maui, Hawaii*

I thank Aurora you for her deep and compassionate listening. She has a very special gift and I feel grateful to get to connect and experience it. I was able to be more honest with myself about my feelings and needs in my relationship with a very close friend with a life threatening illness. My opening up with her brought us closer together. TheQuest also enhanced my meditation experience, which was really great. They go together very well. —*Paula Mantel, Owner/Educator/ Producer, Discovery Learning Systems, Honolulu, Hawaii*

My work and life has really changed and continuing to change because of working with Dr. Ariel. On top of that I have felt really seen by her which has encouraged me to come out more with who I am in the world, something most others cannot do for me since they are not where I am, and don't understand. Her style of counseling resonates with me because it feels very organic to me, creative and natural in working with the psyche and what wants to be seen, acknowledged, transformed, and that our beings want this and know how to do it with help and encouragement and love. This has been an incredible door for me, and my clients are really benefiting. It is helping me to become who I am and what I am here to do. I'm feeling rather teary now with gratitude for divine guidance in meeting Dr. Ariel and the serendipity of life when we open to spirit. —*Lisbeth Walters, Rolpher and Cranial Sacral Practitioner, Columbus, Ohio*

The tools Aurora shared about in her TV interview are so simple, flow easily and have helped me already. I sent an Email about her work to others, and several of us have instantly benefited. The arrangement of her process was much easier than others I've tried. Maybe it is just time for things to be easy. I especially was touched that Aurora allowed the interviewer to be a facilitator, as this shows others that even amateurs can assist healing. I was also impressed that she allowed herself to be the subject. This sends a great message that healers need healing too. I commend her for that openness. —*Libby Coulter, Maui*

I feel lighter... I loved the process! I have been thinking so much about everything I experienced! Many thoughtful doors have opened and I love the unfolding. It has been helping to shape the way I think and feel about my loves in my life and the lesson they bring. —*Elli Clauson, Special Ed Teacher, Aspen, Colorado*

AURORA JULIANA ARIEL PHD

TheQuest

Healing Journal

Healing, Inspired Music, Books & Audio CDs

By #1 Bestselling Award Winning Author, Aurora Juliana Ariel, PhD

Earth 2012-33: The Ultimate Quest - Vol 1
How To Find Peace In a World of Chaos

Earth 2012-33: Time of the Awakening Soul - Vol 2
How Millions of People Are Changing Our Future

Earth 2012-33: The Violet Age - Vol 3
A Return to Eden, The Regenesis that is Birthing a New World

Earth 2012-33: Oracles of the Sea - Vol 4
The Human Dolphin Connection

TheQuest Self Healing System
TheQuest book, Healing Journal, and 7 Step CD

The Indwelling Spirit
An Illumined Pathway to Freedom, Enlightenment and Peace

Sacred Knowledge Collection CDs
Exploring the Afterlife; The Soul's Journey; Journey Into the Future

Healing Music For An Awakening World CDs
12 Healing Music Journeys by Aurora, Bruce BecVar & Krystofer

The Healing Power of Love CDs
7 Divine Healing Transmissions

Renaissance of Grace
Aurora's World Music CD with Bruce BecVar

Gypsy Soul, Heart of Passion
Gypsy World Music CD by Bruce BecVar & Aurora

River of Gold
New Age Music CD by Bruce BecVar and Aurora

AVAILABLE IN BOOK & MUSIC STORES WORLDWIDE

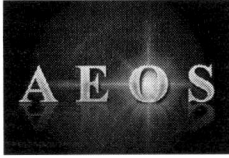

A New Frontier In Multimedia Arts
Inspired Music, Books, & Films

Publisher: AEOS, Inc.
PO Box 433, Malibu, California 90265
Ph: 310-591-8799 Fax: 413-521-8799
Email: Info@AEOS.ws
Website: http://www.AEOS.ws

Art Direction by Aurora Juliana Ariel
Cover & Interior Design by Aurora Juliana Ariel
Interior Master Design by Kareen Ross
Editing by Aurora Juliana Ariel, PhD
Dr. Ariel's Photos by Christian Cooper, Monique Feil

TheQuest Healing Journal
Copyright ©2012 by Aurora Juliana Ariel, PhD.

TheQuest is a cutting edge Counseling Theory and Practice, comprehensive body of knowledge, and complete Self Healing System with tools to heal an ailing humanity. It is the hope of the publisher that it fulfills its mission in reaching everyone it is meant for across the planet.

TheQuest is a proprietary trademarked Healing System. The publisher and author of this material make no medical claims for its or TheQuest use. This material is not intended to treat, diagnose, advise about, or cure any illness. If you need medical attention, please consult your medical practitioner.

Printed in the USA

FIRST EDITION
Library of Congress
ISBN 978-0-9847571-4-5

Dedication

TheQuest
is my legacy to my children,
grandchildren, humanity and a world in need of healing.
It is a saving grace, a healing salve,
and a miracle in the darkest hours.
May it fulfill its purpose
in setting humanity FREE
to fulfill their Highest
Destiny Potential

Contents

Introduction

As so often is the case, Dr. Ariel's personal challenges catalyzed her on the quest that is now changing lives worldwide. Her story speaks to the human spirit who rises from the ashes, overcomes every obstacle, seeks to find meaning in each trial, and translates life challenges into an offering for humanity. She has suffered what many suffer on Earth and come through victoriously, proving a way for people to restore their lives no matter what they've been through. She says, "The pain people carry not only burdens the mind and infects one's perceptual reality, it eventually etches itself upon the physical body causing illness and aging. Aging is not natural. It is simply the accumulation of life's hard hits. To heal the cause of aging, illness, and other dire conditions, you must heal your deep-seated wounds, fears, pain, and trauma. Otherwise, they will adversely affect your life, limit your passion, creativity and joy, and cause you to feel old before your time."

My mother's search for the cause of suffering and a cure began when her mother became seriously mentally ill when she was 19. Standing by her mother through 23 hospitalizations, she sought remedies to alleviate her mother's suffering, helping her to have a more quality life. Another powerful catalyst came at 33, when my mother had two heart attacks within 6 months and was told she had an incurable heart condition that could debilitate her quickly to death. Willing herself to live, she entered a healing path that led her deep into the psyche to unlock the causes behind her illness. Her landmark discoveries from this personal healing journey as well as the countless people she's helped, gave her a profound understanding of the psyche, tools to heal an ailing humanity, and a cure she is now gifting the world in TheQuest.

The immense obstacles she faced over many years helped pave a way that is helping lives all over the planet. With TheQuest Self Healing System (book, Healing Journal and 7 step CD), people can gain mastery over their psychology, heal their addictions and patterns, and live healthier lives. They can emerge from devastating experiences unscathed with the underlying cause healed. They can attain a level of self mastery relatively unknown in this world, live in their Authentic Selves more often, be positive and proactive, making the wisest choices, and bringing their creative expression and unique gifts to our present planetary equation.

Upon meeting Dr. Ariel, no one would ever imagine what she has been through. Her carefree spirit, youthful appearance, and love for humanity demonstrate the healing power of TheQuest. Like many valiant souls before her, she translated excruciatingly painful experiences into a victorious story and offering for humanity. It is this commitment and unswerving devotion to a higher purpose that helped her forge a gift for the world out of her own struggle. Her Life is a testimony that every issue can be resolved, every pattern healed. Seemingly incurable conditions can be changed. Dr. Ariel has paved the way.

Mariah Brown, Daughter of the Author, Maui, Hawaii

Part One

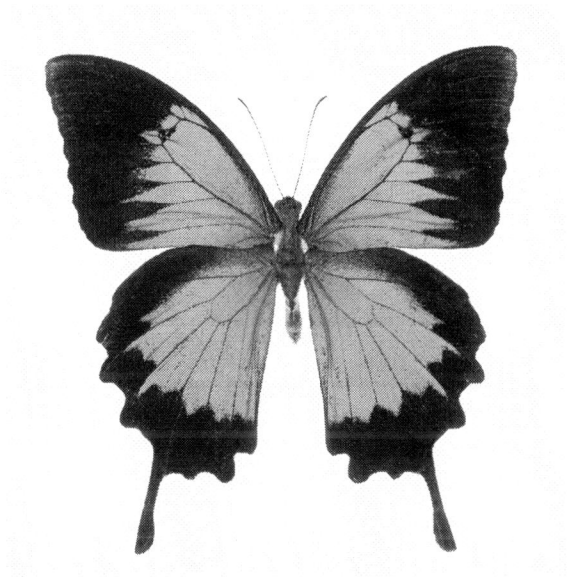

TheQuest
Self Healing System

Through the
mists and silvery veils,
our Illumined Self shines through.
We feel it when we soar with creativity, share love,
feel quiet and at peace, or rejoice in the Wondrousness of Life.
Then, the effervescent energy of LIFE abounds all around us.
At sad moments, we must lift up our heads and remember...
our present trials are but mists rising from the deep,
reflective of inner wounds that are ready to heal.
We are not our wounds or the scarred remains
of the happy child we once were.
We are the Joyous One
who dances free of all encumbrances
and who lives within us, whole and complete
no matter what we pass through.
Do the deep inner work that is calling and
rise like a Phoenix, inspired, ennobled in your Truth,
like the butterfly from the chrysalis...
step FREE!

TheQuest Healing Journey

Over many years of pioneering work in the psyche, I found the cause of suffering. Working on the most impossible cases, I made landmark discoveries that brought an end to the mythology around pain that has plagued our world. I developed a cutting edge Healing System that has changed my life as well as many others. I am excited to hand you the knowledge I've gained. With TheQuest tools, you can completely heal and transform your life. The 7 steps are designed to help you move quickly through your issues, gain a greater understanding of what you have been going through and why, and help you to make the wisest decisions for your life.

One of my most exciting discoveries was finding that when we heal our life, we change our destiny. We do not need to reap the outcome of our family patterns or societal conditioning. We can step free and live the life we were meant for. We can fulfill a higher purpose rather than be relegated to a program dictated fate. When you have the right tools, nothing can stop you and I've proven the way.

In this Healing Journal, I will be laying out the 7 step Self Healing process that can take you from upset to peace in minutes, unveiling the secret formula to gaining greater mastery over your psychology and life. I will show you how easy it is to be in control of your emotions, patterns, and addictions rather than continuously run by them, and how you can live more often in your Authentic Self, which is always peaceful, positive, and proactive. This is the miracle consciousness that allows synchronicities and magic in your life.

From this vantage point, you make wise decisions and take positive action steps. When you do this, you are actualizing your full potential and fulfilling your highest destiny. This is very different than fulfilling the fate dictated by unconscious patterns, which unfortunately is the norm on Earth. By dong this inner work, you can gain a comprehensive understanding of your shadow (unconscious patterns), and how this powerful Life Mastery Path can assist you in realizing your dreams and highest aspirations.

Change is possible, but the knowledge that could set you free from your challenging circumstances, financial constraint, health issues, painful relationship, or addictions has been hidden to this time. It is only in recent history that the first pioneers began a trek into what I call the 'Last Frontier,' which is the uncharted realms of the psyche.

My own journey into the deep recesses of the human psyche has given me a comprehensive understanding of why people suffer and how easy it is to become free of conditions that have forever held people in their grip. I am excited to now be releasing this body of knowledge to the world.

TheQuest Healing Journal takes journaling to a whole new level. Instead of simply writing out your feelings and becoming more aware of your patterns, you will be able to resolve every issue and heal every pattern that arises and begins playing out in your life. With the companion book, *TheQuest: Heal Your Life, Change your Destiny,* you will have all the knowledge and tools you need to continually change the challenging conditions in your life. As you transform your life from within, you will be able to inspire loved ones to do the same. in this way, families and communities around the world can be served.

The 7 step process will guide you safely into a greater understanding of yourself and your psychological makeup. It will assist you to go deep into the heart of your pain, frustration, or anxiety and heal the patterns that are causing your present life challenges. When you do this deep inner work, you find the answers to why these things are happening in your life so you can change them. The 7 steps are easy to apply and is an extremely effective way to extricate you from even the most challenging situations. Deep seated fears can easily be released, anger and rage transformed, and violence or cycles of being abused can be stopped.

The reward of TheQuest work is greater understanding, compassion for yourself and others, happiness, a renewed passion for life, and inner peace. You will find with this Self Healing System, every issue can be resolved, every pattern and addiction healed. You can change the conditions in your life while actualizing your full potential.

This book brings a healing remedy to every situation. As you do the 7 steps, you will find that TheQuest work is powerful, life changing, and profound. If you apply the training in *TheQuest: Heal Your Life, Change Your Destiny* book and use TheQuest Healing Journal to master the 7 step self healing technique, you will become a master of your life in a way that you never dreamed possible, because you will have effective ways to deal with your Shadow as it arises. You will begin living a life that you never imagined was possible, uncovering the true Authentic Self beneath the patterns, as session by session you excavate your the Lost Self and reconnect with your True Identity.

You will find that you are a Spiritual Being having a limited and many times challenging human experience. Having undergone an amnesia that has blocked the memory of who you truly are, TheQuest work can become an exciting journey of self discovery and self empowerment, gifting you a mastery once thought unattainable.

We all have adopted programs that have us believing we are less than we really are, that we are bad, wrong, ineffectual, not good enough, wanting, not lovable, valuable, or have no worth. These misinterpretations lie at the core of all our personality dysfunctions and are behind our life problems.

Restoring ourselves to our Divine Nature is an essential element in TheQuest work, so we can more fully embody the truth of who we are. When we do that, we realize our highest Destiny Potential and fulfill a Divine rather than human plan. That is when life get's exciting!

CHAPTER TWO

The Secret Formula

TheQuest is a breakthrough healing technology that has been time tested with great success on a host of applications like stress, heartbreak, addictions, abuse, anger, violence, low self esteem and more, and on numerous subjects including people from all walks of life, children, teens and youth at risk. It has made a difference in the lives of addicts, abusers, people with health and other serious conditions including anxiety, depression, suicidal tendencies, grief, and trauma, and children and adults who were abused or had great losses. It has successfully healed a wide range of personality traits and dysfunctions. I continually see complete healing and transformed lives from this work and miracles happen all the time.

One miracle took place at my first Life Mastery Training Course in Aspen. I gave a woman a counseling session that took her back into forgotten memories where she had been severely abused. The next day she called me very excited saying a life long debilitation had been healed.

She writes, "I had pronated knees since I was a little girl. Continually aggravating the condition through a very active and full life, it became a life long affliction. By 25 years old I had to stop running, a great passion in my life! I also loved to ski, hike, and bike, but my knees would get so sore that my lifestyle was greatly hindered. At TheQuest Training in Aspen, I had the opportunity to work with Dr. Ariel. In my session we traced a pattern back to early childhood where I had suffered severe abuse. As we unlocked and healed the pattern, I felt a tremendous release. The very next day I was working out at the Aspen Club gym when, looking in the mirror, I noticed my legs were straight. My trainer came over and could hardly believe his eyes. The condition was healed!"

Her condition was a direct result of a wounded inner child, who having been violated and betrayed by someone close to her, had contracted into a protective posture that literally reformed her legs and made them turn inward. When the inner child was healed, she felt safe enough to trust again and was able to open fully. Immediately the condition that she was holding in place dropped away and her legs straightened out. They no longer needed to turn inward to protect her.

I see this all the time with physical conditions that many believe must only be treated on the physical level when the true cause is found within. When you work on this deeper level, you not only change the condition you are facing, you eradicate it from your future. By healing the cause in the past, you stop the pattern in the present, and prevent its return in the future.

One woman came to me in great pain. She was a yoga teacher who had suffered with a hip problem for months. No amount of rest, massage, or other outer methods would relieve it because the cause needed to be found inside her. The Inner Aspect (Subconscious Personality) that was holding this condition in place needed her full attention before she could release the physical condition. After one session, this woman was surprised to find that she was no longer in pain. We had gotten to the heart of her condition by tracing it back to her early childhood and the beliefs she had taken on. Her Inner Aspect then released the pattern and her physical body immediately followed.

A client was on his way to the chiropractor one day. He was in serious pain with his hip out. I could see that it was about two inches out from where it should have been. We began looking more deeply into what this was about and that led us into the Seven Steps. Twenty minutes into the session, I witnessed his hip miraculously move back into place. Needless to say, there was no chiropractic visit that day. We had gotten to the heart of the problem and the condition was healed.

A woman with a severe case of emphysema came to me when she was first released from the hospital. After the first session she no longer needed her oxygen bottle. When she went to see her doctor, he was very surprised at her unexpected return to health and took her off her medication. After two sessions with me, her doctor could not believe she had quit smoking. He had been her doctor for the thirty years she had smoked and twenty of those years he had witnessed her trying to quit. Our work together simply got to the reason why she was smoking. Once we healed the part of her that needed to smoke, she was free of the addiction and cravings.

When the lungs are afflicted, there is a story of grief that is usually tied in. In this woman's case, she had lost her ranch in a foreclosure, her father and her dog had died, and she had gotten a divorce all within a year. Soon after, she landed in the hospital. By getting to the heart of her grief and healing the parts of her that were 'ill', she was able to quickly return to health. Had she not done this deeper work, she may very well have fulfilled her illness's death sentence.

A greatly significant piece to this work is how it can change lives so dramatically. When we are released from patterns that drive us to be a certain way, we can live a life that is more in accord with our True Nature. One example was a teen in Aspen who was a troubled at risk youth. He was using drugs and alcohol and had been arrested five times. He was on probation and was continually in trouble at school.

He began coming to our weekly Teen Forum on his own with some of his friends. My son, who was the same age, inspired him to get a private session from me. In that session, I found that this beautiful boy not only had a bleak outlook on life, but a very dark future. He literally could not see anything beyond further arrests and getting into trouble. He had been estranged from his alcoholic mother and lived with a verbally abusive father who used cocaine and other drugs. His self-esteem was low and his self-confidence shot. A bright future was beyond this teen's comprehension.

Our session went deep into the cause behind his acting out and healed it. In that moment, his future changed. By the end of the session he became passionate about exploring a career in marine biology and said he was committed to doing better in school so that he could get into a better college. That was the day his arrests and trouble at school stopped. His father saw a huge change in him and was surprised to find out that his son was attending our Teen Forum on his own. He called to thank me and told other parents about it who he thought should send their teens.

This boy's court appointed Youth Zone counselor was so amazed by his sudden and complete turn around she wrote, "When meeting with a court-ordered youth, I noticed an enormous shift in his attitude and responsibility in a very short period of time. So I asked him 'What has happened to cause you to mature so quickly?' and that's when he told me that he was in a program for teens that was making a huge difference for him. I have not seen such a huge internal shift in a youth like this in a very long time. My interest in the TheQuest Teen Forum came from seeing results, not from hearing about the program. This is fantastic work!"

Sometimes the outer shift I see is miraculous, at other times the individual must go through a series of sessions to unlock the complete puzzle to a life challenge. This becomes a journey of self-discovery that is incredibly empowering. I see this many times with serious illnesses like the incurable heart and other conditions I have had, and with people who have addictions or conditions like cancer. The psyche (the soul) is not seeking the cure of a moment. It needs time. It wants a complete lifestyle change from the inside out and to have that, it must first release the patterns that are directly related to the old lifestyle and way of being that brought the illness on.

There is a chemical process that takes place when we are imprinted with human programming that changes the very nature of our physical body. That is why you can trace every challenging condition to its origin within the psyche. To heal a serious illness or debilitating condition, the process many times takes a series of counseling sessions supported by restructuring the lifestyle to foster health and well being, which can include products and modalities to help release the disease and restore the body.

Serious conditions, whether an illness or other physical condition, must be addressed on this deep level otherwise it may be cured or resolved in the present, only to return in the future. You want to heal your life challenges on the deepest levels, getting right to the core. By irradiating the root cause of your condition, the physical aspect can more easily be transformed.

Dr. Wayne Topping of the Topping International Institute found that when individuals work with their personal psychology in a constructive and effective way, they experience deeper levels of well being, happiness, and peace. Dr. Topping's work was part of my early foundational training. It gave me the understanding that there was a deeper cause behind my "incurable" illness, which inspired my journey within to find what was really at the heart of my condition. His landmark research into emotions and their effect on physical organs helped me trace what was behind my heart condition and the two heart attacks I had within six months. This led me to the heartbreak that had caused my illness, an important key on my journey to health.

Our challenges are opportunities for growth and learning. They set us on a journey we might never have embarked upon. Fearing the worst, we access an inner strength that might not have been there before. Being overcome by challenges, we find skills we didn't know we had. Facing death, we come to appreciate life more reverently.

When we are dying, we want to live. The moment we face our darkest hour, we turn to the light. When we're held in the grip of an illness or debilitating physical condition, we seek health. When we are constrained by our finances, we seek freedom and relief. Our inner self kicks in and takes command. That is the physics of this soul journey. When you have the secret formula to unlock your life situations from within, challenges that once seemed insurmountable or conditions that felt unchangeable are easy to shift.

Many times a client will come to me feeling they can no longer take it. They've tried everything to no avail. When I tell them, "Don't worry, it's a piece of cake!" they look at me in disbelief. This work is so cutting-edge that most people on the planet cannot imagine that there is relief like this available. They suffer on with their addictions, they feel relegated to being overweight, they can't imagine living without tension and stress.

One client wrote, "My heart is so open and full from this work. Being gently led through the deepest, darkest places leaves only gratitude, love and freedom. In every session we come quickly to the taproot of the issue, create safety for its exposure and transformation, and watch the magic with awe as the entire tree is healed. This work helps me feel so purposeful. I am proud to be a human, finally. The tools that Dr. Ariel uses for healing are pure magic, like laser surgery for the soul. The operation is fast, relatively painless and totally effective. People would not choose to live with pain if they knew this was available."

Each session is an incredible journey of self discovery taking you to the heart of your life challenges and healing them from within. When the pattern is healed, you emerge victorious and feel empowered and free. It is then you realize how affected you were by your patterns and how they had held you in their grip. Sometimes you are being suffocated by your subconscious patterns and you don't even know it. You've lived with them so long they have become a normal way of life, you don't even realize you are living in a prison.

There is a freedom and peace that is available to you but you will never realize it until you begin delving deeper into what is really going on in your life and face how you really feel about it. When you systematically extricate yourself from everything that is holding you back and limiting your creative expression, you set yourself free from what could have been a life sentence.

A businessman and Real Estate Broker in Denver wrote, "After years of being in and out of therapy I had changed my life very little but after four sessions with Dr. Ariel I was a new person. I had come to the first session a skeptic, but by the time we were done I was totally amazed by the amount of healing that took place. I had been hitting my head against the wall, not getting any movement in my years of therapy. Traditional therapy had only scratched the surface, whereas TheQuest dove right into the root of the issue, uncovered the truth, and healed that aspect of my inner self. The sessions have been the most powerful events in my life! I'm finally free of the unhealthy part of myself that was holding me back for years. I never thought transformation like this was truly possible. I'm no longer a victim of the past and my emotional traumas have been set free. I have my life back! I've made more progress in a few sessions with Dr Ariel than I have in years of therapy."

Recently I heard from him in an email. He said, "Since we worked together, a lot changed in my life. I married the woman of my dreams and it has only gotten better. Now we have a little daughter. This was all made possible because of yours and TheQuest work. Thank you, from the bottom of my growing heart!"

While miracles are commonplace with TheQuest, some conditions require that you take time to unlock each piece of the puzzle. In that way, you gain a conscious awareness of a complex pattern that is responsible for your challenging condition. Your life can miraculously change in one session, or you may be on a healing journey that can take months or even a year. Whatever the time period for your complete release, it will be an interesting and life changing journey.

By applying TheQuest Self Healing System, you can change your life. You can step free of addictions, lose weight and live a healthy life. You can heal the causes behind your anxiety and be released from tension and stress. You can create more harmony in your relationships. When you tend to the deeper conditions in your life, there is a self-nurturing aspect that is very comforting. You begin relaxing and finally, you sink into an exquisite peace. Your life situations are resolved and you are released from their prison. Very quickly, you come to understand what has been behind the challenges you have faced. This helps you have compassion for yourself and others.

We're in an age of miracles where everything can change in a twinkling of an eye. With TheQuest Master Keys, we can turn everything around. We can quickly extricate ourselves from human programming and step free to realize our full potential. We can bring our Authentic Self into the equation and fulfill a higher destiny.

As you apply TheQuest Seven Steps, miraculous changes will begin taking place within you. Every area of your life can change. As you break free of the confines that left you feeling limited and living less than your potential, you awaken to who you truly are behind all the personality traits and patterns. You begin realizing your value and worth, and are able to bring forth your unique talents, expertise, knowledge and gifts to make a difference on the planet.

CHAPTER THREE

TheQuest
Life Mastery Path

Mastering the Art of Self Counseling is an important key to Inner Peace. The more adept you become at this, the more you will be your Authentic Self, experiencing a sense of freedom, happiness, fulfillment, and joy. The key is to do TheQuest 7 Steps as issues arise, rather than suppressing your upset or wrestling with your feelings while being completely overcome and run by them. So, how can you masterfully traverse challenging conditions and still maintain a level of composure and your creative edge, deal with the phantoms that rise without warning from the dark recesses of your psyche and hold to a sense of equanimity and grace? How can you manage your anger while maintaining loving relationships?

Understanding this dilemma, I was inspired to release my work to the lay person rather than just giving it to practitioners as is normally done when a Counseling Theory and Healing Practice is developed. I realized that if I distilled my practice into a Self Counseling Technique that was easy to apply, it would give people the ability to deal with their issues in a timely way. I was excited by the idea that many more people than I could personally assist would be able to experience profound healing and be able to do this inner work in the privacy of their own homes.

For years I have done my own Self Counseling sessions. This work is empowering, taking me through some very challenging times. During Dark Night periods, people around me would be amazed. How could I go from being that upset to calm, peaceful, and clear in less than an hour! This was an area of mastery no one had heard of.

It was my son, Aradeus, who insisted I translate TheQuest counseling technique into seven steps, so that he could give the formula to the teens in the weekly Teen Forum he had initiated in Aspen, which he and I were co-facilitating. So, I wrote them out and what we saw was amazing! The kids loved it and some of them actually ran with it and changed their lives! One 15 year old, who attended a progressive school, was able to use TheQuest Journal of Self Counseling sessions to fulfill one of her course requirements. The school was so impressed they invited Aradeus and me to present this work to her whole class.

One week she came to the Teen Forum with an incredible story. She shared how she had spent time with a dear friend over the weekend who was suicidal. I asked her, "How is he doing now?" She said, "Fine. I took him through the 7 steps!" This amazed me! I saw then how so many people can be helped with this process.

During that time, I was invited to present TheQuest to two classes at Aspen High School where I took the teens and their teacher through the Seven Steps. The response was incredible. In one class, the teacher was extremely concerned about how I would be received. He said, "This is an unruly bunch of kids. They don't pay attention and they can be extremely rude." Imagine his surprise when the kids in his class were riveted on what I was sharing the whole 90 minutes, and not only that; they all did their Self Counseling with the Seven Steps, many of them sharing their process with the class after each step.

At one point, the supposedly "coolest" kid in the school went to the blackboard, drew his Inner Aspect and began writing his feelings on the board while the other students supported him with suggestions. The teacher was stunned! In his letter of recommendation the teacher wrote, "I have to admit that I was a bit skeptical how this would play out to a group of 20 or so usually somewhat inattentive high school students. Both classes were surprisingly attentive and interested in what Dr. Ariel presented. The fact that she held everyone's attention with something that was somewhat foreign to all of these students and she had all the class thank her as she left for the day and others asking for more, told me that she was on the right track with the work she has dedicated her life to. I also followed along with the class in the exercises she had designed for that day and was amazed at the insights that were provided to me in so brief a period of time."

In the past, a Counseling Theory and Practice would be given to practitioners to apply with their clients. In this way, the community was served, but it didn't address the greater problem, that humans had no control or mastery over their psychology and therefore were unable to be wise stewards of their lives. Tossed by the sea of planetary challenge, it was a rare individual that could steer his or her ship quickly into clear waters. Most people are completely overwhelmed by challenging life circumstances. They do not have the tools to traverse them with skill. To handle situations, many will bury their feelings and then will later become ill or will "lose" their tempers, ruining relationships or chances of advancement at work.

As I've watched the miracles of TheQuest in my own life and the lives of my children, clients and students, I've wanted to share it with the world, to give it "to the people." That is why I always educate and train my clients while I am working with them. I have such a strong sense that it is important to pass on this knowledge, to help people understand their psychology, and to give them the tools to change their lives.

One client in Hawaii wrote, "Gone are the days of long drawn out traditional therapies. With TheQuest I have found a way to heal and transform any pattern or history from ancient to present times. I have found a new sense of purpose in life with each healing of the darker aspects of myself, a greater love for all that I am. TheQuest allows me to address issues as they come up and access the core of the issue to transform it all in one session! Aurora's dedication to the healing arts has empowered me as a wife, mother, businesswoman, healer, and human being." It is responses like these that have kept the fire burning inside of me to bring this work to everyone it is meant for!

TheQuest Life Mastery Path is simple. The moment that an issue is up, when you feel distraught, angry or upset, it is time for TheQuest Self Counseling. The sooner you get to this work, the faster you will have your issue resolved. In this way, you shorten the time of misery, and return to the harmony and peace of your True Nature quickly.

If you want to traverse your life and display the greatest mastery, you must address your issues as they arise. Following the Seven Steps, you can facilitate your own Self Counseling process, tracing your feelings to the part of you that is calling for attention and healing. By applying the Seven Steps, you can move yourself quickly from upset to peace, while healing a pattern that has contributed to the challenging condition in your life.

Preparing for your Self Counseling session is important. In chapter 5, I give you steps that will help you create a safe space that will allow you to go to the deepest levels in your healing and in Chapter 6, I lay out TheQuest Seven Steps. As you learn this Art of Self Counseling, it is best to use a journal. In this way, you will be able to stay on track with your session from beginning to end and have a record of the healing that took place to review in the future. Doing this in a journaling format allows you to track your progress and is a profound way of supporting yourself through your life journey. Once you master this technique, you can also do the Seven Steps as a self-guided inner process.

Becoming proficient in this work, you become a Master of your Psychology, working on important elements in your psychological makeup and healing them as they arise. With each Self Counseling session you feel more whole and complete. As you restore each imperfect facet of your personality to its innate design, you tap into the awesome power of your Authentic Self and its ability to manifest its high vision in your life. No longer run by your unconscious patterns, you heal your issues and transform your patterns as they come to your conscious awareness. By practicing the Art of Self Counseling in a timely way, you make the wisest choices for your life and fulfill your Highest Destiny Potential.

CHAPTER FOUR

Self Counseling With TheQuest

This Healing Journal can become your best friend, someone you come to each day with your heartfelt desires, life intentions, insights, and revelations, and who is there to help comfort you in times when you are in pain. Incorporating TheQuest work into your journal is a powerful way to have the greatest growth and advancement from each life situation. In this way, you can accelerate your journey and become powerful, clear and directed as your steer your life course from your Authentic Power rather than limited self.

TheQuest Self Counseling is a way to go to the heart of life conditions, unlock them from within, and heal them for the last time. When we you this inner work, the outer world changes around you. As you learn to be more peaceful, the world will reflect your inner peace. This is how peace can be restored on Earth, one person at a time, and why I feel excited to offer TheQuest as a remedy for a world in travail.

This powerful, cutting edge technique can change your life, because it works directly with the subconscious aspects in charge of your challenging life situations, transforming them from within. Mastering the Seven Steps, you become adept at freeing yourself from challenging circumstances. When you apply this technique, you have found a Master Key to Inner Peace.

Each time you free yourself from the grip of upset feelings you return to your True Nature, the part of you that is always calm, centered, and peaceful. When you learn how to set yourself free from every challenge and resolve your issues quickly, you begin to experience an exquisite joy in your new found freedom. Dealing with challenges quickly and effectively, allows you to do more of the things you enjoy in life and you are happier when you do them You have a new passion for life, because you are operating from your Authentic Self, free from debilitating emotions or low self esteem.

In each Self Counseling session, you are able to understand the challenges you've encountered, realize the great value and growth they brought to your life, and see how they assisted you in having more compassion for yourself and others. In finding a way out of each dilemma, you not only become a master of your life, you have developed a gift of greater awareness you can now share with others. In overcoming life challenges in this masterful way, you gain a unique insight into your psychology and healing patterns becomes an exciting journey of self-discovery and awakening.

How To Work Your Self Healing Process

When you feel upset or when you have an emotional response to something that happens in your life, it is time to do TheQuest Self Counseling. When you deal with your feelings on this deeper level, you resolve your issues quickly and you gain the clarity and insight needed to handle the situation effectively.

Self Counseling is an essential element of TheQuest Life Mastery Path. It provides the tools that allow you to gain control over your emotions and heal facets of your psychology that are sabotaging and holding you back. By working your Self Counseling process as issues arise, you are able to return to a clear calm place where you can direct your life course more effectively.

TheQuest Seven Steps are designed to help you get to the heart of your upset feelings and resolve them. When strong feelings arise, it is important that you feel your emotions fully, refraining from self-judgment. Being with your feelings helps you get in touch with what is really going on inside and will help you access the part of you that is feeling that way. Tending to this upset in a timely way is important.

You may feel that the situation warrants a strong emotional response, and it is natural you would feel that way. But when you are upset, you are not in the natural balance and flow of your True Nature, and actions and decisions fueled by these feelings can be destructive. It is extremely important to turn within when you get upset, because your feelings will lead you to a place inside that is calling for attention and healing. Ignoring your feelings will only delay the deeper resolution and healing that is available to you.

Your feelings are allies. They draw your awareness within to an upset aspect (subconscious personality) that was wounded or colored from the past. The event that triggered your emotional response activated this inner part of you. As its feelings come to your awareness, you are able to work with it.

What is important to know is that an Inner Aspect is never activated unless it is ready to be healed. Each time you are upset or become aware of a pattern, it is an opportunity for you to step free from a program that has limited or held you back. It is a call to change your life in an important way at the perfect time for your soul advancement.

When you do this inner work, the shift that occurs can be profound. By listening to your feelings and trusting this inner process, you are able to release yourself from the core pattern in charge of your situation and move to the next level of conscious awareness.

When you emerge clear and centered, you are a commanding presence that is in charge of your life and destiny. You are no longer tossed on the sea of life without a rudder or clear direction to guide your way. You have returned to the clarity of your True Nature and to your authentic power.

The Seven Steps

In **Step One**, **Identification,** it is important to step back into a "witness" point of view once you have fully felt your feelings. In this way, you can see the part of you that is upset and work with it directly. Many people believe they are the upset part, so it is hard for them to distinguish that only a part of them is feeling this way. The truth is, there are many facets to the personality. You can have many conflicting parts. For example, you might feel very angry, but at the same moment you may also think the situation is not worth getting upset about. You may have a part of you that hates someone, while another part feels guilty and ashamed for feeling that way. One part may be tired and worn out, while another part feels like it must drive you onward.

Stepping back and centering in your Authentic Self, the neutral observer that continually witnesses your life from a calm clear bastion of peace, allows you to work effectively with the part of you that is upset. You want to help it get to the truth that will resolve the issue from within. This is the moment when you take the reins of control. You have moved your conscious awareness away from the upset part to the wise minister and healer governing your life destiny. From that place of power, you compassionately guide the Inner Aspect (the part of you that is feeling the emotional upset) through the seven steps to its complete resolution and healing.

Time is of the essence. It is best to do TheQuest Seven Steps within 24 to 48 hours of an upset, otherwise, the feelings recede and it is harder to identify and work with the part of you that is up for healing. You want to work with this part, because it has a direct relationship with the challenge you are facing.

The Inner Aspect will feel like a victim, but it has helped create the problem. It is the saboteur and the one that drew in the challenge. Its programming dictated its fate. You are there to free it.

In **Step Two**, **Influence,** you find how the subconscious aspect has been affecting you in each area of your life. It may be shutting you down or constricting you. It may be a volcano that explodes, ruining your core relationships and destroying your self-esteem. Whatever its affect on you mentally, emotionally, physically, and spiritually, whether it is creating an illness, undermining your health, destroying your peace of mind, or causing immense stress, allow it to share with you openly. If you judge the Inner Aspect, it will not only go away and hide from your conscious awareness, but the condition will remain unchanged, while the pattern continues to create similar situations in your life until you are finally ready to deal with it.

In **Step Three**, **History**, you trace the history of the pattern back to the original wound. Let the Inner Aspect guide you through its painful past, reviewing the histories it brings to your conscious awareness. Keep your mind quiet. Don't try to remember the past or to think up the answers to the questions. Just relax and let the Inner Aspect show you.

You want to steadily guide it back to the originating incident. Following the history into the past is important for your Inner Aspect, because it allows it to see where its pattern stemmed from and how it was reinforced in your life. To make sure you have reached this originating point in time, ask the Inner Aspect if this is where it first took on the pattern.

Think of this process as if you are lovingly taking the hand of someone who is very wounded and hurt. You are following them down into the caverns of the psyche to what could be a very dark and scary past for them. Your love, compassion and caring is the key. The Inner Aspect will trust you to know what is best and will allow you to guide it to its complete healing. This is its journey to freedom and the result for you and the Inner Aspect will be enlightenment and peace.

In **Step Four, The Truth,** you will discover the point in time when the Inner Aspect took on the beliefs and self-judgments that created the pattern. This is a very important step for the Inner Aspect because this is where it was imprinted with misinterpretations about itself. These self-judgments are usually something like, "I am unworthy of love. I don't matter. I am not good enough. Something is wrong with me. I am bad." The Inner Aspect may feel ruined, damaged, or stained. It will have influenced your life from this vantage point, permeating your conscious reality.

Core beliefs become patterns that are etched in time. These reoccurring patterns play movies that reinforce beliefs like "I am not good enough," and will continue until you go to the heart of the belief system and change it at its core. You also pick up beliefs that are passed down through your family lineage by family members who are struggling with their own life conditions. These beliefs can be, "Life is hard. Suffering and pain are a part of life." Religious beliefs similarly traverse family lines such as, "I am a sinner that must pay for my sins." There is a host of beliefs and self-judgments that have plagued the human race and created suffering as a way of life on earth. We all have similar core beliefs, but the way we got them is our unique story.

Once the Inner Aspect has become aware of this imprint, you help it trace the effects forward to the present time, seeing how they influenced your life. You are now able to see the real reason for your life challenges. This is an elemental key to understanding life conditions and how they originate in the psyche, first as beliefs, and then reoccurring patterns. When this takes place in the session, there is an awakening that helps you see your responsibility in the equation. It is not that we consciously will "bad" things to happen to us, it's just that our core beliefs form patterns that create the challenges in our life. The good news is that once identified, these beliefs can be changed and the patterns healed. Once this takes place, the outer condition will shift.

I included Step Four in TheQuest Counseling technique because of its significance in bringing conscious awareness that on some level we do create our reality and because it is our creation, not the will of an outer deity or accounting system, we can change it. When you fully understand that the reoccurring patterns in your life are born from these beliefs and how they have adversely affected your life, you hold an important key to your freedom.

Once your Inner Aspect is fully aware of how your inner programming was being reflected in your outer reality, you gently guide it back to the originating incident to see what the truth is.

Are the beliefs and self-judgments it took on accurate?

The Inner Aspect will find that it is innately pure, not bad or evil at its core. It is lovable, it is good enough, it is worthy of love. This is when a powerful inner shift occurs. You have gone down into the core wounding and are now emerging with the Truth. The part of you that was stamped with this pattern and scarred from the painful life experiences, is now free to fulfill its highest potential. Though it may have felt ruined, tainted, or destroyed, it will be released from the fate dictated by the programming. In that moment, a complete history is being laid to rest and a new future is beginning to dawn on your horizon.

It is in **Step Five, Higher Purpose,** that you gain an overview of why the pattern served you and what the Inner Aspect wanted to accomplish. This helps you understand the greater purpose behind the challenges you faced and how they were important for your life. This is a powerful step that takes victimhood out of the equation, because it frees you from the sense that you are a victim to your fate.

You begin to see the perfection in everything you've gone through and why it was important for you. You are uncovering the truth, overcoming the pattern, and freeing yourself from false beliefs that created a false identity. As the cause of your pain is healed, the pattern will no longer be playing out in your future. You will be free!

Your subconscious patterns provide life circumstances that challenge you in unique ways, and each serves you in accomplishing something important. You may have become stronger, you may have more insights into human nature, or you may have a greater compassion and desire to help others. They help forge your destiny and assist you in finding your True Purpose.

Once you see how the pattern served you and what gifts you gained from it, your Inner Aspect will feel complete. It will now be ready to let go of the pattern and be a positive, rather than challenging, support in your life. The Inner Aspect will no longer need the pattern to fulfill its goal in challenging you for your own betterment.

In **Step Six**, **New Intention,** you ask your Inner Aspect to give you a new image of the new intention it has for you. You have it place the new image next to the old one, so you can see the difference. The new one will be radiant, powerful and strong, while the old one will be wearing the affliction it was overcome with.

In **Step Seven**, **Transfiguration,** when your Inner Aspect is ready, you have it step into and merge with the new image, bringing all the wisdom, learning, and growth it gained, and letting go of all detrimental aspects of the pattern, including the pain, self judgments, and beliefs it took on. In that moment, a powerful inner transformation takes place. The Inner Aspect is now free, enlightened, and clear. You have transformed the shadow to light, your upset to peace, your pain to joy, and restored a flawed facet of your personality to its innate design.

This Sacred Alchemy of the Soul is a deep inner process that alchemically changes the very nature of your life experience. It undoes the past and transforms the future. It restores you to your

True Self, the part of you that is always in peace.

With this understanding of the subconscious and the knowledge that you can skillfully heal and transform every challenge in your life, you no longer need to live with painful dynamics or feel burdened about your past. You can step free from memories that have plagued you.

By healing your patterns, the conditions of your life give way to allow a more enlightened, harmonious, and fulfilling existence. The Truth of who you are shines through. The baggage you've carried for so long is gone. Jewels of Wisdom have replaced painful histories as your past is reframed. You understand and are at peace.

CHAPTER FIVE

Creating Time for Your Healing

One of the essential elements in TheQuest Life Mastery Path is to create time and space for your healing. This is time for you. Make it special. You journaling process should be a joy, gift you a retreat from the world with quality time all for you.

Create a Safe Space: When giving yourself a counseling session, it is important to first prepare a space where you will feel comfortable. Turn off the phones and make sure you will be left undisturbed. Lighting a candle, burning incense, creating a centerpiece with flowers or healing stones can be very comforting. Add your own special touch to create the atmosphere most inspiring to you. You can find a serene nature setting, sit in a beautiful garden, or do the Self Counseling at the beach. Get creative! This is a powerful experience that is deeply empowering and restoring.

TheQuest Self Counseling Journal: Journaling your process can be empowering. It allows you to trace the history of your Self Counseling sessions and see where and when you addressed and healed a pattern. You begin to see how powerful this work is in changing your life circumstances and altering your future. The more creatively you express in your journal, the more you will be inspired to bring your issues there.

This is Sacred Time: A time to express yourself fully and to heal parts of you that were wounded in the past. This Self Counseling process is nurturing to the wounded spirit, allowing the deepest reflections to take place. It can restore you quickly and help you come through the most challenging experiences unscathed. As the integration occurs and positive life changes take place, many powerful revelations and timely insights can come forward. Writing these in your journal along with all your victories adds a tremendous depth to your life passage.

Centering yourself and then beginning with a clear intention or prayer for the session is very powerful. You can ask that the greatest healing take place within the deepest levels of your psyche, your family line, and in humanity, being specific about the upset or pattern you want to resolve.

TheQuest Self Counseling Technique: You will find TheQuest Seven Steps in the next chapter. Simply follow each step until your Inner Aspect is completely healed and transformed. To do this, you must first get in touch with your emotions. Once you have done that, you can step back into a neutral observer position to work with the part of you that is upset. The key is to get a clear visual image of the Inner Aspect during Step One. Once you are able to identify the upset aspect, you can then take it through the Seven Steps.

It is important to be kind and compassionate with the Inner Aspect rather than judgmental. Criticism of your feelings and the part of you that is upset will only drive it away from your conscious awareness. If that happens, you won't be able to work with it. Not feeling safe, it will recede back into your psyche until a future time when it is triggered again. Meanwhile, its pattern will continue to bring dysfunctional relationships and challenging situations into your life.

Think of the Inner Aspect as a child who needs your care and attention, even though it may appear in adult form. Many Inner Aspects received their encoding in childhood, but they may appear older when you begin working with them.

You want to heal each troubled aspect of your psyche as it comes into your conscious awareness because it is the one holding the code to the subconscious programming that is responsible for your outer challenge. To unlock this code and reprogram it, you must work on it directly in the subconscious where the patterning occurred.

Where to Begin: At the top of your journal page, write the date so that you can trace your positive life changes and victories to the specific session and pattern you healed. Then begin with Step One, writing, "1. Identification." Follow the instructions, writing out the answers and continue this format throughout the counseling session. Feel free to draw your aspect as it goes through the different changes during your session.

Remember: Emotions are your allies. They appear at the perfect time to lead you into the psyche where you will find the next pattern ready to be healed. Once you become proficient in this work, you will be able to do the Seven Steps effortlessly as issues arise. Addressing your issues and healing your inner patterns will become second nature.

- Always treat yourself and your Inner Aspects with love and respect. The more compassionately you embrace an Inner Aspect, the more willing it is to share its story with you. This will help you traverse the dark regions of the psyche, bringing healing to even the most challenging aspects.

- If you ever feel stuck, or the aspect is not responding, go back to the previous question and continue working with it until all the important information is gathered and it feels good about going to the next step.

TheQuest Seven Steps

When you apply TheQuest Self Counseling technique, you are working on a deep unconscious level. The inner shift you will undergo will then ripple out to positively affect your life. This can bring miraculous results to challenges that have felt unchangeable or insurmountable. Remember, every issue can be resolved and every pattern healed. You can change the conditions of your life! Leaving your issues unaddressed or ignoring your feelings can have detrimental effects. Doing your Self Counseling in a timely way can bring immediate relief and give you ability to more effectively handle what you are facing in your life.

Step One: Identification

1. Review what you're going through, or a condition or illness you are facing, and what you are feeling. Allow yourself to feel your feelings fully, then write these feelings down.

2. Next, move back into your Authentic Self, so that you can get a clear visual image of the part of you that is feeling this way and that has the condition, giving it loving attention rather than criticism or judgment. Visual imaging is important. *Once you can see an Inner Aspect, you can heal it.*

3. Draw a picture of your Inner Aspect and then write down everything it is feeling. If the upset is a result of what happened with another individual, you can draw them as well, so you can get a clear visual image of this dynamic.

An Important Key: Your dynamics with others are a reflection of what is happening inside of you. The sooner you move your attention away from what is going on between you and the other person, the quicker you will resolve your issues and be able to effectively deal with the situation. The other person's unconscious words or actions supported you by triggering a deep pattern or wound that is ready for healing. If you are dealing with an illness, financial constraint, or other challenging situation, include that in the image, showing how the Inner Aspect is being adversely affected.

Step Two: Influence

Now it is time to begin working directly with your Inner Aspect. Ask the Inner Aspect how it has been affecting you on all levels (physically, mentally, emotionally, spiritually) and how it has been influencing your life (relationships, health, career, finances.) List each area and then write down the answers.

Step Three: History

Ask the Inner Aspect to show you the history of similar feelings and experiences all the way back to where the pattern originated and then see what was taking place at that earliest time. Write the highlights.

Step Four: The Truth

1. Find the self-judgment and core beliefs it took on from that earliest experience. (I was unloved, therefore I am unlovable. I'm not wanted, I don't matter, I'm not good enough, etc.)

2. See how these judgments and beliefs influenced your life, tracing the pattern forward to the present time.

3. Go back to the original incident and see if the judgments and beliefs were really true, asking the Inner Aspect, "What is the truth?" Have the Inner Aspect review each judgment and belief and update it with the new realization.

Step Five: Higher Purpose

1. Ask the Aspect, "Why was this pattern and the experiences it created important for me? What did you want to accomplish?"

2. Once you have received a positive answer ask, "Do you feel you have accomplished that?" If the answer is no, take the Inner Aspect back through some of the previous questions until it has accessed everything it needs to move on.

3. Then ask, "Do you feel complete with the pattern?" The answer should be yes.

4. Next ask, "What would my future look like if you chose to continue the pattern instead of healing it today?" Remember to keep writing the answers in your journal, stopping to tune in to your Inner Aspect as you go along.

Step Six: New Intention

Ask the Inner Aspect what its intention is for you now, and ask it to give you a new visual image of what that would be and look like, placing the new image beside the original one. Draw or describe this new image in your journal, listing the new intention beside it.

Step Seven: Transfiguration

1. When it is ready, have the Aspect merge with the new image, retaining all the learning, growth, wisdom, and knowledge it gained, while dissolving all aspects of the pattern that no longer are serving you. This should include all the anger, upset, and pain it was feeling and all the self-judgments it was holding.

2. Once complete, ask "How will my life be different now that you've been healed and transformed?" Draw or describe the transfigured Aspect.

3. Ask the Transformed Aspect, "What action steps should I take to support this session?" Write those down. Having a copy of them will remind you so you can stay on track with supporting the inner shift that has occurred.

Integration: You have just gone through a very deep and powerful inner process. Allow yourself time to anchor the new information. You may want to do some additional writing, listen to inspiring music, or just have some time alone in nature.

This quiet time is important for you to integrate what you have been through. It will allow you to more fully understand the pattern you healed and what it created in your life. You can emerge from this process with a new sense of empowerment and compassion for yourself and others. Remember to journal your experience and make notes relating to your session when your life changes in the future.

Remember to use the Seven Steps whenever you feel upset or are facing a challenging life situation. Use this counseling technique before you work on issues with your mate, colleague, child, or friend. You'll be a lot clearer and more able to come from a centered, compassionate place, where you will be able to listen as well as share your experience in a loving way.

Feel free to share TheQuest with loved ones and friends. The more people that adopt Self Counseling as a part of their lifestyle, the more a true and lasting change in relationships can occur, positively affecting the consciousness of the planet. With such a dramatic shift away from victimhood and blame, the world can transform very quickly, allowing peace to replace suffering as a way of life.

Share Your Experience: I'd love to hear about your experience with TheQuest and to receive testimonials for this work if you feel it has benefited you. You can email your experience, testimonial, or personal story to me at: Info@IOAH.org

CHAPTER SEVEN

Unveiling the Authentic Self

There are many positive by-products from TheQuest work. You will find, as you do your self counselling in a timely way as issues arise, you will be in your Authentic Self most of the time. Clear, directed, positive and proactive, you will be dealing with life challenges masterfully, showing great skill as you avail yourself of the opportunities they bring.

By uncovering your True Self in each session, you will feel empowered by the truth of who you really are, and you will more easily recognize when you are acting out of who you are not, the programmed wounded self. Programs that used to run will quickly fall to the wayside, allowing the Authentic Self to take command of your life. Myths of the past will be laid to rest as you adopt a new attitude based on the truth - that you are worthy, lovable, and deserving. When you know you are worthy, you create a life that reflects your self-esteem. You feel supported from within and your path becomes less arduous. You stand for what is your highest good and have clear boundaries. You live an exemplary life. It is then you build your foundation upon the Principles of Peace.

Forever, humanity has been out of touch with the Authentic Self and that is why the world looks like it does and why there is so much suffering. To reclaim that Lost Self is an exciting journey of self discovery, self empowerment, self fulfillment, and self actualization. It is a coming of age, a maturing in the divine sense. In realizing the truth of who you are, and daily reclaiming that reality in every area of your life, you become a bastion of freedom and peace. You are a shining example to others, who are inspired to follow the enlightened way you live. Consciousness is catching. So can many, in this time, rise into their full potential selves and help create a better world.

As you become more attuned to your Inner Self, you can access its wisdom and keep a record of its inspiration in your journal. Dipping into Authentic Selfhood, many realizations take place. You become insightful and wise. Serenity and peace is another sign you are in your Authentic Self. You live from a higher vantage point.

I call this the Miracle Consciousness, because it is the Authentic Self that does all the magic in our life. It draws in all the right people and circumstances, and synchronicities become daily occurrences. This way of life is so magical. Allowing the Inner Self to lead is so much easier than struggling on in our patterns, trying to control our life when most things are beyond our control. TheQuest has been my greatest ally and has made a huge difference to my life. I would not live without it! I hope you will allow it to do the same magic in yours.

Part Two

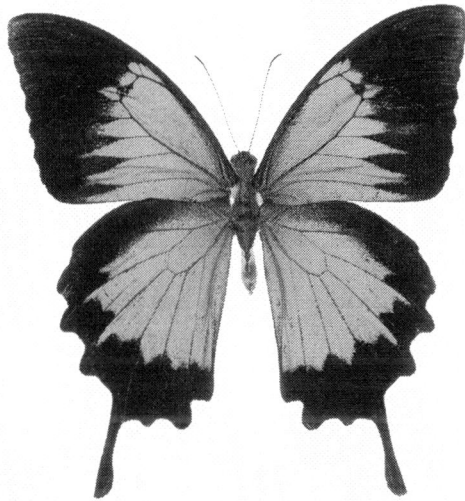

About the Author
Products, Programs, and Services

About The Author

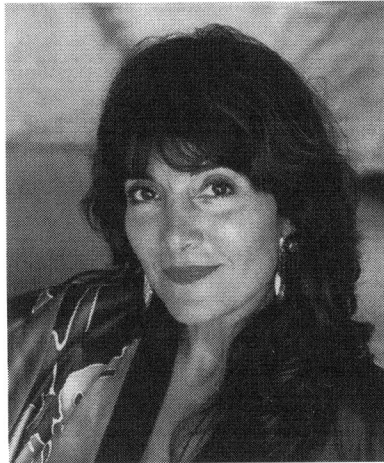

Whether its pioneering work in the psyche, bringing out her landmark discoveries in global conferences, writing books, leading TheQuest Trainings, or expressing her musical talents, Aurora Juliana Ariel possesses the proverbial Midas touch. Her brand of alchemy is the sacred sort, yielding a gold one can only discover within. Pioneering doctor and scientist, author and musician, entrepreneur and producer, mystic and healer, Aurora is a Renaissance woman for the New Millennium.

A Humanitarian Futurist with an extraordinary heart and offering for humanity, Aurora Juliana Ariel, PhD has dedicated her life to creating a better world through three vehicles focused on positive planetary change: the Earth Vision Foundation (Lemuria Rising - Earth Vision Center Project), Institute of Advanced Healing (bringing out TheQuest worldwide) and AEOS (a new frontier in multimedia arts in healing, inspired music, books and films).

Creator of TheQuest (a breakthrough psychological healing system), #1 Bestselling Author, and Award Winning Author of the Earth 2012 Series, she is a Pioneering Doctor and Healer whose research and work have given her a profound understanding of the psyche and the tools to heal an ailing humanity. Working with countless individuals with miraculous results, she has made many landmark discoveries bringing a new understanding to our present planetary equation. She speaks eloquently of the significance of this time in Earth history and the challenges before us, bringing a timely remedy and insights inspiring people worldwide to make a difference. She holds over 35 certificates and degrees in advanced healing methods as well as a B.A., M.A., and PhD in Psychology. She is also a Kahuna, the successor of Hawaiian Kahuna, Shaolin Grandmaster Pang.

All of this pales, however, in comparison with the work Dr. Ariel has done on herself and her work directly in the psyche with countless clients over many years, resulting in the development of her Counseling Theory and Healing Practice, TheQuest, which she calls the 'Ferrari Model' of Inner Healing work.

A Spiritual Scientist in the Laboratory of the Soul, Dr. Ariel took her vast body of knowledge and went deeper on her own quest for healing. She discovered a way out of pain and suffering, a transformative technique that changed her life and brought tremendous healing to her clients.

Dr. Ariel has taken TheQuest to the next level and offers it as a complete Self Healing System that includes her powerful seven step Self Counseling Technique. Her reason for bringing it to the people, rather than simply releasing it to professional counselors is simple. She wants to bring healing to a world in desperate need.

Dedicated to positive planetary change, Dr. Ariel sees this period on Earth as a time when we, as a humanity, desperately need to uncover and heal the subconscious patterns she believes is at the heart of the dire conditions we are presently facing. When we accomplish this, we become the peaceful, loving, happy individuals we were meant to be and the world changes around us.

For more information about Dr. Ariel, her work and products see: http://www. AuroraJulianaAriel.com. To support her efforts, you can make a tax deductible donation to the Institute of Advanced Healing at: http://www..IOAH.org. Your donation can also donate TheQuest: Heal Your Life, Change Your Destiny books or Complete Self Healing System (book, Healing Journal, CD) to rehab centers, prisons, hospitals, health retreats, safe houses for the abused, addiction, abuse, and youth at risk programs, or place of your choice. Your donations are greatly appreciated!

TheQuest

TheQuest is a revolutionary breakthrough Counseling Theory and Healing Practice that includes a complete Self Healing System developed by Dr. Ariel after years of extensive research and work. It is designed to bring timely knowledge and a missing piece to rehab centers, prison reform, addiction, youth at risk, 12 step and other programs, greatly increasing their success rate.

For practitioners, it is a way to move your clients quickly from upset to peace, and to help them quickly resolve deep issues, step free of limiting and self sabotaging patterns, addictions, and dysfunctional personality traits, and realize their greater potential.

For the layperson, it is a way to gain greater understanding and mastery of your psychology, empowering authentic self-expression and creative fulfillment.

For couples, it is an essential ingredient in conscious relationship, where each person works with their own psychology as issues arise. Greater harmony and clear communication can exist when the focus is on resolution through loving, compassionate interactions.

The Institute of Advanced Healing

In 2000, Aurora Juliana Ariel, PhD founded the Institute of Advanced Healing, a non-profit organization in Hawaii, to bring forth her life's work, TheQuest, which includes TheQuest Trainings, Classes, Counseling Sessions, Support Groups, advanced healing products and services.

Dr. Ariel developed certificate-training programs and set up a model chapter in Aspen, Colorado in 2005 to be duplicated around the world by graduates of TheQuest Master Counselor and Spiritual Leadership Training Courses. She has successfully worked with youth at risk, addicts, abusers, and the abused, people with serious illnesses and trauma, and a host of dys-functional personality traits and life conditions with tremendous results. She has given classes to teens at High Schools, released TheQuest to the public on her websites, TV, radio, support groups, and via her Ask Dr. Aurora Column, and is now training people in her seven-level Certificate Training Courses provided through the Institute. For more information see http://www.IOAH.org and http://www.TheQuest.us.

The Human Dilemma

The work at the Institute of Advanced Healing has a very clear focus: to bring TheQuest to a world in dire need. The subconscious programming that has created the human condition with its propensity for misery and suffering must be healed. People worldwide need to understand their psychology and learn how to become masters of their destiny, rather than victims to their fate. The cause of suffering must be healed for the world to begin to reflect the noble ideals that are encoded in the hearts of humanity.

When people are engulfed and entrapped in their human patterns, a higher destiny is never fulfilled. Instead, the destiny that plays out is from this programming. The degree that the higher nature, which Dr. Ariel calls the 'Authentic Self,' can express through the individual, the more the person will be able to experience a higher awareness and ability to attain a greater mastery over their life circumstances. Presently, this is very rare on Earth. Even in the spiritual communities of the world where the greatest trainings and highest information is attained, there is a continual dysfunctional aspect to people's lives, because the subconscious patterns are not being addressed. They are being suppressed or spiritually bypassed, while they continue to work their havoc.

It has long been believed that people cannot change their personality traits or heal their addictions. The best that can be done is for individuals to understand their patterns and strive to overcome them. But this method does not work because physiologically the limbic system, the part of the brain that is activated under stress in what has been called the Fight and Flight Syndrome, is different from the area of the brain where the will and determination is found, which is in the frontal lobe. Therefore, under stress, the individual will revert to Fight and Flight, and the subconscious pattern will begin running. They will move into survival and seek substances or run other addictive behaviors to alleviate suffering. Physiologically, the blood will recede from the frontal lobe impairing will and therefore control.

When the deeper patterns have not been addressed and healed, people will understand their addictions and strive to stay sober or substance free, but if they undergo a series of life stresses, it will be easy for them to fall off the wagon. This is because the subconscious has been left out of the equation.

Currently, because the deeper work is not being done, there is only an 8% success rate in rehab centers and addiction programs. The programs today help strengthen the individual's resolve, but do not provide a complete healing. TheQuest Seven Step Counseling Technique provides the 'missing piece,' which can greatly increase the success rate at these centers and with people suffering from addictions of every kind.

A Breakthrough Technology

Understanding the human dilemma and being concerned that psychologists today normally only scratch the surface when working with clients, thereby keeping people coming for sessions for years without any real movement, Dr. Ariel developed a way to move people quickly through their issues and heal their underlying patterns. Her revolutionary method provides a complete resolution, healing, and breakthrough in each session.

If you would like to sponsor or support Dr. Ariel's work and the Institute's mission to bring TheQuest to communities throughout the world, donations are tax-deductible and greatly appreciated. To make a donation, please go to http://www.AuroraJulianaAriel.com, http://www.IOAH.org, or http://www.TheQuest.us

TheQuest Life Mastery Path

When you understand your psychology, you have greater control over your life circumstances. As you master TheQuest tools and learn how to heal every condition from within, you have a greater command of your destiny. Your Authentic Self is given room for a fuller creative expression in and through you and a new passion and excitement about life returns. You wake up looking forward to each new day and what amazing things will happen next. Unexpected events and synchronistic meetings increase resulting in key alliances with like-minded people for a greater purpose. Life takes on a sweeter quality, as you know you are fulfilling a sacred destiny. TheQuest Life Mastery Path training is available in TheQuest courses, providing you with the tools and knowledge of how to free yourself from every pattern and condition that has limited you, kept you feeling disempowered, burdened, or held back, so that you can realize your full potential.

Heal Your Life, Change Your Destiny

When you heal your life, you change your destiny. It is as if you are defying a powerful law like gravity. For the human patterns within you are creating a different reality than the Life your True Nature would give you. Clearing the way for this Authentic Self to lend its wisdom and power to your life, allows you to fulfill a higher destiny.

TheQuest Counseling Sessions

While Dr. Ariel is largely on sabbatical focusing on writing, appearances, and training individuals worldwide, she is from time to time available for personal sessions and for shorter personalized training programs. These are weekly or bimonthly sessions over 6 months to 1 year that include Life Coaching and Counseling sessions along with personal training in TheQuest Life Mastery Path. Dr. Ariel is also available at times for personal 7 - 14 day retreats, where her focus is completely on you and your optimum health and well-being, and for Total Life Intensives where every area of your life is addressed and transformed.

TheQuest Training

Dr. Ariel holds TheQuest Certification Training Courses all over the world. If you'd like to sponsor her in your area, receive counseling sessions or life coaching, or receive certification as a Life Coach and Counselor, please email her at: info@aeos.ws. TheQuest Training consists of three level certificate courses. Levels 4 - 7 are for those who want a career as a Life Coach, Counselor or Spiritual Leader in the Organization.

Become a Certified Life Coach and Counselor

TheQuest Life Coach and Counselor Certification Course provides an in-depth study of psychology in a format that is experiential, life changing, and empowering. These highly informative trainings, within a compassionate caring environment, can be taken via phone from anywhere in the world.

Each course is unique per the student and their current life challenges and is, therefore, a journey to the heart of these conditions where they are completely healed and transformed, returning you to Authentic Self awareness. You master tools to heal self sabotaging patterns, addictions, personality traits, and dysfunctions, deal effectively with health and career issues, and transform challenging relationship dynamics. In this way, you transform and empower your life while learning how to help others.

As you learn how to clear a pathway to the Authentic Self and its inner wisdom, you begin to give it more power in your daily life and to fulfill your higher Destiny Potential. By mastering your 'shadow,' you learn to live in the Miracle Consciousness. This is when you begin living a Miraculous Life.

TheQuest Life Coach and Counselor Training is a one-year (or accelerated 9 month) certification course working directly with Dr. Ariel each week. Highly experiential in its application, this program gives you the life mastery skills, knowledge, and tools to become a Master Life Coach and/or Counselor, with the ability to practice anywhere in the world. Doctors, Psychologists, Health Practitioners, Life Coaches, and Ministers may qualify for the accelerated training program with Dr. Ariel for TheQuest Counselor Certification.

TheQuest Programs
Healing Lives, Changing Destinies

Total Life Transformation Program

Life Coach & Counselor Certification Course

Counselor Certification Course

Miracle Weight Loss Program

Relationship Healing

Addiction Release Program

Brain Chemistry Balancing

Women's Empowerment Program

After Rehab – Maui 21 Day Retreat

Maui Rejuvenation 21 Day Retreat

In-depth information on all programs and products
can be found on the following websites:

http://www.IOAH.org
http://www..TheQuest.us
http://www.AuroraJulianaAriel.com

TheQuest Self Healing System

TheQuest Book, Healing Journal & 7 Steps CD

TheQuest

Heal Your Life, Change Your Destiny

TheQuest
Heal Your Life
Change Your Destiny
7 Steps To Radically Transform Your Life
A Breakthrough Self Healing System

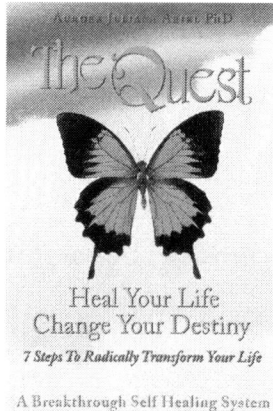

A Breakthrough Self Healing System

"This book will ignite a Revolution In Consciousness
so powerful, it could restore Peace on Earth."

"People would not choose to stay in pain
if they knew this was available."

In this ground breaking book, Dr. Ariel unveils her breakthrough Healing System, the 7 Master Keys to Inner Peace, and a powerful Life Mastery Path. She demystifies the psyche like no other work has done and provides tools to quickly resolve issues, restore harmony in relationships, master your psychology, and heal the scars from your painful past.

Through years of pioneering work in the 'uncharted realms' of the psyche, she made many landmark discoveries, uncovered the cause of suffering, and developed a cure that could change the destiny of the planet.

Distilled into seven powerful steps, TheQuest is designed to accelerate a personal and planetary transformation that could help end suffering on Earth. Inspiring a Journey of Self Discovery that is empowering and life changing, TheQuest unlocks the Secret Code to your True Identity and provides a Key to Actualizing your Full Potential.

TheQuest
7 Step Self Healing System

TheQuest
7 Step Self Healing Technique
How to Heal Your Life & Change Your Destiny

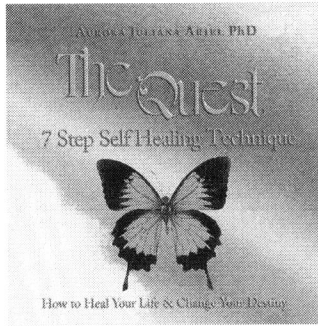

A dynamic element in TheQuest Self Healing System
to help you heal your life and change your destiny

"This CD will be the breakthrough many have been waiting for,
giving people a way to heal their lives in the privacy of their homes
with tools they can use for every challenging situation."

"People would not choose to stay in pain
if they knew this was available."

In this CD, Dr. Ariel unveils the 7 Step Self Healing process she developed that can help you quickly resolve every issue, heal every pattern, change every challenge and emerge from every situation victorious.

Gently, she guides you through the 7 steps in a healing journey of self discovery, self empowerment and self actualization. As you journal your inner process, insights, revelations, understanding and compassion for yourself and others emerges. Self judgments fall away as well as misconceptions and misunderstandings. You emerge feeling empowered, clear and directed, a whole piece to your family dynamic and inner patterning resolved.

'TheQuest session with Aurora unblocked a subtle but powerful limitation in my life. I am grateful to her for her work and for her safe and gentle way of being.'

-Jack Canfield
author of 'Success Principles' and
co-author of the 'Chicken Soup for the Soul' Series

Part Three

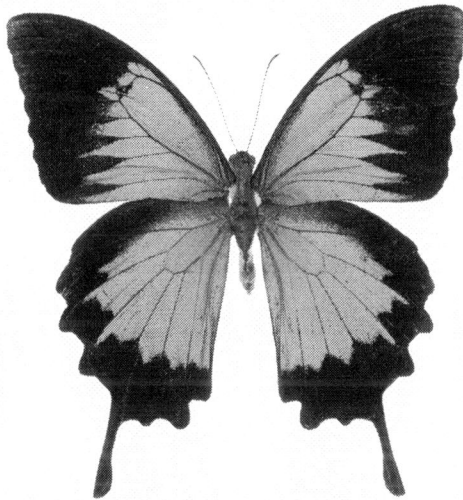

TheQuest Healing Journal

TheQuest 7 Step Self Counseling Technique

When you apply TheQuest 7 Steps in your journal as issues arise, you are working on a deep unconscious level. The inner shift you undergo will then ripple out to positively affect your life. This can bring miraculous results to challenges that have felt unchangeable or insurmountable. *Every issue can be resolved and every pattern healed. You can change the conditions of your life!* Remember, leaving your issues unaddressed or ignoring your feelings can have detrimental effects. Doing your Self Counseling in a timely way can bring immediate relief and give you the ability to more effectively handle what you are facing in your life. Follow these 7 Step:

Step One: Identification

1. Review what you're going through, or a condition or illness you are facing, and what you are feeling. Allow yourself to feel your feelings fully, then write these feelings down.

2. Next, move back into your Authentic Self, so that you can get a clear visual image of the part of you that is feeling this way and that has the condition, giving it loving attention rather than criticism or judgment. Visual imaging is important. Once you can see an Inner Aspect, you can heal it.

3. Draw a picture of your Inner Aspect and then write down everything it is feeling. If the upset is a result of what happened with another individual, you can draw them as well, so you can get a clear visual image of this dynamic.

An Important Key: Your dynamics with others are a reflection of what is happening inside of you. The sooner you move your attention away from what is going on between you and the other person, the quicker you will resolve your issues and be able to effectively deal with the situation.

Application: The two images you see described on the page are no longer you and the other person. They now represent your own Inner Aspects. Because they have gotten your attention, they are now ready to be healed. In this way, the other person's unconscious words or actions supported you by triggering a deep pattern or wound that is ready for healing. If you are dealing with an illness, financial constraint, or other challenging situation, include that in the image, showing how the Inner Aspect is being adversely affected.

Step Two: Influence

Now it is time to begin working directly with your Inner Aspect. Ask the Inner Aspect how it has been affecting you on all levels (physically, mentally, emotionally, spiritually) and how it has been influencing your life (relationships, health, career, finances.) Write down all the levels and the answers. (MENTAL, EMOTIONAL, PHYSICAL, SPIRITUAL, HEALTH, CAREER, FINANCES, RELATIONSHIPS)

Step Three: History

Ask the Inner Aspect to show you the history of similar feelings and experiences all the way back to where the pattern originated and then see what was taking place at that earliest time. Make sure you are at the earliest time and write the highlights.

Step Four: The Truth

1. Find the self-judgment and core beliefs it took on from that earliest experience. (I was unloved, therefore I am unlovable. I'm not wanted, I don't matter, I'm not good enough, etc.)

2. See how these judgments and beliefs influenced your life, tracing the pattern forward to the present time.

3. Go back to the original incident and see if the judgments and beliefs were really true. It helps to go over what was really happening. Ask the Inner Aspect to update each judgment and belief with the new realization.

4. Next, Self Forgiveness can be a powerful healing salve. Place one hand on your heart, the other on your stomach and say, "I forgive myself for judging myself as (or, I forgive myself for believing…)" going through all the judgments and then stating the Truth.

Step Five: The Gift

1. Ask the Aspect, "Why was this pattern and the experiences it created important for me? What was the gift? What did you want to accomplish?" The Inner Aspect provided you with a 'vehicle of experience.' Have the Inner Aspect review and see what you gained from the pattern. What was the learning and growth?

2. Once you have received a positive answer, ask, "Do you feel you have accomplished that?" If the answer is no, take the Inner Aspect back through some of the previous questions until it has accessed everything it needs to move on.

3. Ask the Inner Aspect, "Do you feel complete with the pattern?" The answer should be yes.

4. Then ask, "What would my future look like if you chose to continue the pattern instead?"

Remember to keep writing the answers in your journal, stopping to tune in to your Inner Aspect as you go along.

Step Six: New Purpose

Ask the Inner Aspect what its intention is for you now, and ask it to give you a new visual image of what that would look like, placing the new image beside the original one. Draw or describe this new image in your journal, listing its New Purpose.

Step Seven: Transfiguration

1. When it is ready, have the Aspect merge with the new image, retaining all the learning, growth, wisdom, and knowledge it gained, while dissolving all aspects of the pattern that no longer are serving you. This should include all the anger, upset, and pain it was feeling and all the self-judgments it was holding.

2. Once complete, ask "How will my life be different now that you've been healed and transformed?" Draw or describe the transfigured Aspect.

3. Ask the Transformed Aspect, "What action steps should I take to support this session?" Write those down. Having a copy of them will remind you, so you can stay on track with supporting the inner shift that has occurred.

Integration: You have just gone through a very deep and powerful inner process. Allow yourself time to anchor the new information. You may want to do some additional writing, listen to inspiring music, or just have some time alone in nature. This quiet time is important for you to integrate what you have been through. It will allow you to more fully understand the pattern you healed and what it created in your life. You can emerge from this process with a new sense of empowerment and compassion for yourself and others. Remember to journal your experience and make notes relating to your session when your life changes in the future.

Remember to use the Seven Steps whenever you feel upset or are facing a challenging life situation. Use this counseling technique before you work on issues with your mate, colleague, child, or friend. You'll be a lot clearer and more able to come from a centered, compassionate place, where you will be able to listen as well as share your experience in a loving way.

Feel free to share TheQuest with loved ones and friends. The more people that adopt Self Counseling as a part of their lifestyle, the more a true and lasting change in relationships can occur, positively affecting the consciousness of the planet. With such a dramatic shift away from victimhood and blame, the world can transform very quickly, allowing peace to replace suffering as a way of life.

.